Autoimmune Diseases, Depression and Anxiety

Discovering How to Advocate for Your Health

Cobi Silver MSW

Cover art by Kathryn Huckins
www.kathrynhuckins.com

ISBN: 1495946673
ISBN-13: 9781495946677

Library of Congress Control Number: 2014903782
CreateSpace Independent Publishing Platform
North Charleston, South Carolina

Dedication

In memory of my grandmother, Sherry Kline - Silver, who passed away from multiple sclerosis

To my dear friend Chrisma Crumpton, the strongest person I know

Contents

Introduction

*I*n an effort to provide patients with the tools they need to successfully advocate for their health care, I wrote this self-guided workbook. As a mental health care professional and autoimmune disease patient, I draw from both my work and life experience to offer this unique resource for those struggling with the emotional impact of an autoimmune disease. In five actionable steps, this guide can help you find your voice, and gain mastery of your health care journey.

Each person is unique, and each person who picks up this book will be at a different point in his or her health care journey. The purpose of this basic workbook is to help you discover what you need and teach you how to advocate for yourself. You may not need to go through all the steps; in fact, you may know how to do some of the steps much better than I am able to portray in this book—and that's fantastic. You may find you struggle with certain steps or are unable to apply them to your condition or lifestyle, and that's OK, too. This is your journey, your life; make this book your own. You can go through the steps just to try something different or use the ideas provided to come up with your own ideas. This may be extremely helpful to you, or you may find you are in a different place in your health care journey and just want to pass this book along to someone who could use it more. Wherever you fall in this adventure, I wish every one of you peace, comfort, and healing.

The roller-coaster ride that comes with diagnosis can be overwhelming, isolating, and scary. It becomes easy to just nod your head and agree with everything the doctors, nurses, and social workers say. It's even easier to just go through the motions and do what you're told with the thought that maybe—just maybe—life will go back to normal someday. As the days turn to years and the years pass, it gets harder to go through the motions. You become worn out, tired of telling the new counselor your story because you've already told it to six other counselors or social workers, who faithfully come every time you're admitted to the hospital. You're tired of seeing countless doctors who never really know what the best course of treatment is for you because so little is actually known about autoimmune diseases. Life turns gray, and you walk, more slowly now, one foot in front of the other, trying to smile and be brave so your friends and family won't worry.

As your health deteriorates and you realize that the terrible side effects from the medications are in fact much better than the symptoms you experience without the medication, you feel little pieces of your life begin to chip away. This decision you have to make between a life with embarrassing side effects or a life with painful symptoms consumes you and makes you feel you must have done something to deserve this. All the doctors say they don't really know what caused your autoimmune disease. They say there could be multiple factors. They say it isn't anything you have done wrong. But all you hear is that you are somehow defective.

You feel defeated because people can't see your illness the way they can see that of a patient with cancer who is going through chemotherapy. People don't know about many autoimmune diseases, and they don't understand them. Instead of receiving support and love, you are bombarded with questions, doubts, and confusion. The all too frequent "but you don't *look* sick" can bring you to the verge of tears. You feel as if you have to justify your illness to other people, to plead with them to believe you. You answer the same question over and over again, pushing play on the recorded message you have mastered in your brain after being asked, "So, what *is* lupus?" five million times. You feel bad for getting annoyed and feeling overwhelmed with the questions because the people asking are trying to understand—they are trying to be empathetic. But having to list your symptoms and then defend yourself against the growing number of people who think a cure is as simple as making a change in your diet is draining, mentally and physically. Family, friends, doctors, counselors, and strangers look at you like you're a junkie because you have to take prescription narcotics just to get out of bed in the morning. People don't even give you a chance; they all think you're drug seeking. You feel worthless. You close your eyes and imagine, just for a moment, that people can see the damage that the disease is causing inside your body. Surely if they could see what you look like on the inside, they would not judge you.

Doctors begin to mention to your family that they are concerned for your mental health. Social workers enter your hospital room with information about where you can go to get counseling. But the thought of talking to another counselor now makes you angry. Your disease is something that will get worse with time, not better, and that is a reality many counselors cannot see or understand. You don't feel like being positive because there is no hope for a cure, and slowly you lose hope that your life will go back to normal.

You stop checking your mail because all you get are piles of medical bills and letters from insurance companies stating they are dropping you from the plan you have been paying years for, denying you coverage on a new plan, or promising to cover everything except for anything related to your disease. The financial burden of chronic illness becomes too much; it's too overwhelming to think about these medical bills that will never stop coming. There is no light, and your world feels smaller and much darker.

When you're in this dark, cold place it can feel nearly impossible to get out. You're in the mud, and you feel like you're sinking. No one is hearing your cries for help, or maybe they just don't know how to help.

Fortunately, beautiful things can grow in the mud. They adapt; they survive. The roots of the lotus flower are planted in the mud beneath ponds and rivers. Drowning in mud, beneath water from the very start, the lotus flower overcomes these obstacles, grows through the mud, finds its way to the top of the water, and blooms into a gorgeous flower, colorful and vibrant. Each lotus flower is unique in color, size, shape, formation, and location. Each flower survives given its unique set of circumstances, and each flower makes the world a more beautiful place.

When you're diagnosed with an autoimmune disease, you can feel overwhelmed, stuck in deep mud and nearly drowning like the lotus flower. Living with the circumstances of your diagnosis and the path you must now travel may feel impossible, but if you fight through the thick mud, do your best to swim gracefully to the top of the water, take a breath, and look around, you can see the unique beauty you bring to the world. You may have been planted in hostile, harsh conditions, yet somehow you have learned to adapt and become the most beautiful and vibrant person you can be.

It takes a lot of time and hard work to get through the mud and get your head above water in order to feel as beautiful as you are, but the road you travel to get to that point makes you strong and resilient. It's OK if you're not there yet; it's OK if you can't even picture that point in your journey. For some people it can take just a matter of days, but for others it can take years or a lifetime. Your diagnosis (and prognosis), your life circumstances, your past, your job, your environment, your support system—all of these factors can have an impact on the amount of time it takes you. Just take it one step at a time.

Step One

Understanding Autoimmune Disease with Co-occurring Depression and Anxiety

Autoimmune diseases are basically diseases in which the immune system attacks healthy tissue and cells, causing damage. An estimated 23.5 million Americans suffer from autoimmune diseases, and there are about eighty different types of autoimmune conditions. Recent research has pointed to a link between autoimmune diseases, depression, and anxiety. Though medical and mental health professionals have varying opinions on what causes this, they generally agree that people with chronic illnesses such as these do have a higher prevalence of depression and anxiety.

Some of the clinical data show that the long-term inflammation caused by autoimmune diseases—chronic elevation of proinflammatory cytokines—is responsible for depression and anxiety. Some scientists say that the depression in these patients is caused by signals sent from the gut to the brain. Essentially, any change in the immune system can impact the microbiota in the gut, and these changes can in turn affect the central nervous system. Still other scientists argue that it is the dramatic shift in lifestyle that causes depression for people managing autoimmune diseases. They argue that people who lose feeling in their legs, people who have to now take medication every day, and people who are always sore and tired because of autoimmune diseases are depressed because their lives are more difficult.

Whether the causes are physiological or psychological, or a combination of the two, understanding them is important in order for professionals to more strategically and effectively help those affected. Research now shows that depression can exacerbate symptoms of autoimmune diseases and vice versa, causing the patient to become stuck in a cycle in which each condition triggers the other. The extreme nature of many autoimmune diseases makes it critical that professionals understand how to holistically treat people who manage these diseases—that is, how to provide treatment that addresses both the autoimmune disease and the co-occurring mental health conditions that can cause the disease to become more active.

In order to understand autoimmune diseases and co-occurring depression and anxiety better, I held a focus group and spoke with many people affected by autoimmune diseases. One participant made the following remark, which is helpful in understanding why professionals don't always catch the depression and anxiety that accompanies autoimmune diseases:

> Autoimmune diseases are intense, so sometimes we just want to be strong for everyone else. Let us be strong in front of you, and then let us be weak afterward.

When participants were asked which mental health services are helpful, responses were nearly identical:

> *I think a support group would be fantastic. It would provide us with people we can talk to who can help us and who we can help, too.*

> *There is definitely something to be said about having someone to vent to and that person just listening, and when they say that they understand, you know that they really do understand because they are going through it too, which is comforting.*

The economic impacts of autoimmune diseases are vast. When co-occurring mental health conditions are added to the equation, the economic impact can be detrimental to individuals and their families. Feelings of hopelessness may arise from the feeling of being buried in medical bills:

> *I think a lot of the depression has to do with the financial part of it, too. You know, it's like the bills never stop coming—they just keep piling up, and this will never end. There is no end in sight.*

> *It's the financial barriers that cause a lot of anxiety for me, too. It's like I can go without care and die sooner but still eat and have somewhere to live, or I can get care but be homeless and hungry. Picking the better of two evils. I never win.*

Clearly, something needs to be done. Those quotes are intense, but they paint an accurate picture of what is happening right now with autoimmune diseases, depression, and anxiety.

Now that you have an understanding of autoimmune diseases, depression, and anxiety, we will focus on what you can do to advocate for your health. But before we do, take a moment to think about what inspires you. What are your favorite inspirational quotes? Write them below.

Quotes

_____

_____

_____

_____

_____

_____

Step Two

Discovering What You Need

*P*eople often say that *need* and *want* are two very different things, but that is not necessarily true when it comes to health. Often the two are interconnected. Take, for example, the following statement: "I want to feel better, but in order to feel better, I need an effective medication to manage my condition." In this case, the want or desire is dependent on the need. Now consider another example: "I want to drink a soda, but I need to drink water." In this case, the want is different from the need. When you are working to discover what you need, your needs may overlap with your wants. Try to think of things you could really benefit from. If they happen to fall into both the want category and the need category, that is absolutely OK.

As you can probably predict, I'm going to ask you the classic miracle question. Ready? Imagine going to bed tonight just as you always do, but tonight a miracle happens. When you wake up in the morning, everything in your life is exactly as you would like it to be. What does your life look like? Don't get too carried away here. While it would be nice if a tall, dark, and handsome man (or the equivalent in a woman) magically appeared, for this exercise focus on yourself and the things that would truly make your life more peaceful. If this miracle did happen, would you be happy? Would you be walking? Would you be sitting on the couch, watching *Grey's Anatomy*, house clean, and glass of wine in your hand? You decide.

While a lot of people can think of at least one thing that would improve their life, for some people, picturing things as better can seem impossible. If you find yourself struggling with this step, you can do two things. First, recognize that you are doing great. The fact that you are reading this guide shows that you are trying despite how difficult it is. Before we get to the second, I would like you to search Google Images for "baby animals." Scroll through the images of baby animals for a while, just to clear your mind. When you're done looking at the baby animals, think of a time in your life when things were better. Was it when you were five and you learned to ride a bike? Was it when you were in high school and you went to your first dance? Was it in college? Was it when your first child was born? Maybe it was when you ate a piece of cake or went for a long drive. Think of that time in your life—even if it was only a moment—in which things were better. Keep thinking about that moment. What did you feel? What did you smell, taste, touch, and do? What did that moment look like?

If you would like to answer the miracle question, use the following two pages to write and draw what "better" looks like. Those who would prefer to reflect on a moment when things were better or not as difficult can instead use the following two pages to write and draw that special moment.

Write

Draw

Now that you've spent some time discovering how you would like things to look, let's focus on what you need to do in order to get there.

What do you need? This is an important question that everyone should ask himself or herself. It can be extremely easy to answer, such as, "I need my autoimmune disease to go away." But more often it is extremely difficult to answer, especially if you feel you need five million things right now, and obtaining any of them seems unlikely or impossible. It's important to understand that this question is context based. What is it that you need to help you with your autoimmune disease, your depression, or your anxiety? What is it that you need in order to achieve your "better"?

These are tough questions, particularly when you're not feeling well. The following list of sample needs can help guide your thought process.

1. I need my health care team to listen to and understand me.
2. I need people to stop feeling sorry for me.
3. I need people in my life who understand what I am going through.
4. I need to feel better so I can do better.
5. I need to stop isolating myself.

Do any of those sound like something you need, or is your list completely different? The next page provides you with some space to develop your needs. You can come up with as few or as many needs as you would like—this is your life, and you are the expert.

Brainstorm

Needs

1. _____

2. _____

3. _____

4. _____

5. _____

Have more? Keep going!

Step Three

Talking To Your Existing Health Care Team

*L*et's face it: doctors can be intimidating, and social workers cannot fix everything. The thing is, most doctors, nurses, and social workers really care about people. They truly want to help you be holistically healthy. The difficulty lies in the fact that health care workers (including mental health care workers) see many different people every day, and each person is completely unique. You have your own needs, feelings, sensitivity to pain, interpretation of situations, understanding of conditions—the list could go on forever. The point is, you are unique, and it is impossible for professionals to know exactly what you need unless you are able to effectively communicate it to them. You are the expert in your life. You know your body better than anyone else, and no one can possibly know what it is like to feel what you feel. This is why it is extremely important for you to be your own best advocate.

Understandably, many people struggle with this. It's OK to struggle with becoming your own advocate—and well worth it. Once you master the art of advocacy, collaborating with professionals about what you need becomes much easier.

One of the first steps is using your list of needs. However, putting your needs into words in dialogue with your doctor isn't always easy. Sometimes it helps to humanize your doctor. You might try to sneak in a few harmless questions during your appointment in order to get to know your doctor a little better. When he or she asks about something specific, try to describe the problem, and then insert a quick question at the end. For example, if your doctor asks you if you're experiencing any side effects with your new medication, you might say, "Yeah, my leg sometimes goes numb, and it becomes hard to walk. Has that ever happened to you?" The doctor will likely just give a quick reply and move on. The answer the doctor gives isn't really what's important; it's the fact that you had the opportunity to change the dynamic, even if it's just a little bit. In this way, the exchange becomes more of a conversation and thus less intimidating. You might sneak in a few questions at the beginning of an appointment instead, which also can help to shape the doctor-patient relationship. For example, when your doctor asks, "How are you feeling today?" answer honestly and add, "How about you?" Sometimes doctors will give you short answers that may feel cold, but, again, it's not the answer that matters. By asking your doctor quick questions, you shift the perceived power dynamic in the relationship. You encourage collaboration between you (the expert in your life) and the doctor (the expert of health and medicine). It's important to keep the appointment about you and your health and of course to not cross any boundaries that should be established in a professional relationship, but asking innocuous questions humanizes the doctor and can help you feel more comfortable.

Doing this will not instantly transform your life. Nor will it make it extremely easy to talk to doctors—not at all. But it is an approach worth trying, to see if it fits with your personality and your unique situation. Considering you are the expert in your life, what would work for you? What could you do to collaborate with your doctor? How can you become comfortable with your doctor and find your voice for self-advocacy? Provided below is space for you to work through some strategies of your own. You can brainstorm ideas or make a list of strategies you would like to talk to a friend about. Remember, in this section we are focusing on how to feel comfortable and confident with speaking to health care professionals.

Strategize: How to become more comfortable talking to your doctors and nurses

_____

_____

_____

_____

_____

_____

Brainstorm: Ideas to discuss with a trusted friend or family member

Strategize: How to become more comfortable talking to your counselor or social worker

_____

_____

_____

_____

_____

_____

_____

Brainstorm: Ideas to discuss with a trusted friend or family member

Step Four

Creating Your Support Network

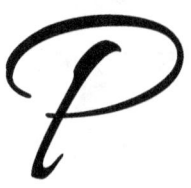eer support groups, in addition to consulting with mental health professionals, are recommended for people with autoimmune diseases and co-occurring depression and anxiety. Focus group participants strongly suggested peer support, as the following comments indicate:

I think it would have been better if someone had told me about how the lupus would affect me. I had no idea, and then—bam! My entire life is thrown upside down, and now I have this condition they are telling me I'm going to die from…but I was healthy yesterday. I think I really just needed to sit down with someone who had been through it before and hash things out. I needed to know what to expect, someone to guide me because this…is intense. There is no end, either. Like with cancer they can say, "Oh, you can beat this." No, that's not the case with lupus. We cannot beat this, we will never win, we will always be lupus patients—and one day it will kill me. That is not something that is easy to accept and not something I really want some counselor telling me, "Oh, you can do some deep breathing, and it will help." It will not help. It will make me frustrated that I wasted precious moments of my now limited life on breathing deep when all I really need is to talk to someone who knows what I'm going through so I can understand it myself.

I agree. It's just different with peers—we can truly understand one another and give real advice without worrying about being professional.

I need a peer support group because I want to be able to call someone at eight in the morning when I'm having trouble getting ready because of my disease—someone I can call when I need help, someone who can give me tips for how to get going.

Peer support networks can look different for different people. A good way to get started is to contact the local chapter of the national foundation for your condition. For example, a person with lupus could benefit from contacting the Lupus Foundation of America and could find local support by contacting the local chapter of the foundation. A person with multiple sclerosis should contact the National Multiple Sclerosis Society and get involved with the local chapter. Sjögren's syndrome also has a national foundation, the Sjögren's Syndrome

Foundation. Google may be the best way to learn about the national support organization for your specific condition or disease. On the following lines, you can record the information you find in your search.

What is the name of the foundation, society, organization, group, or nonprofit for your condition?

_____

What is the name and contact information of someone at your local chapter who can help you get connected?

_____

_____

What upcoming events could you attend in order to meet people (e.g., a walk, a fundraiser, a meet and greet)?

_____

_____

_____

Another way to build a support network is to talk about your disease with other people, whether trusted friends at work or school or family members. When you open up about your condition, people often say something like, "Oh, my neighbor has an autoimmune disease," or, "I know someone with arthritis, too!" You then can assess whether or not that individual would be a good person to try to contact for potential support.

Use the space below to brainstorm other ways you can find people with similar conditions to become your support system:

Below, start developing a list of people you can call when you need support. (Try to include their names and phone numbers, just in case.)

1. _____

2. _____

3. _____

4. _____

5. _____

Having someone to call when you need support or to have lunch with periodically is really the best peer support system. However, I recognize that sometimes depression and anxiety can be debilitating, making it feel impossible to do such things. Fortunately we have the Internet. If you don't yet feel ready to establish in-person peer support connections, but you still want to try to meet people who can understand your condition, online support groups can be great. Google different types of support groups and supportive chat rooms, but be careful about the information you disclose online. Instead of venting all your frustrations and concerns to an anonymous audience online, try using this method as a stepping-stone to establishing in-person supports.

On the following lines, write down some of the support forums or supportive chat rooms you like the most:

1. _____

2. _____

3. _____

4. _____

Step Five

Developing Your Self-Care Routine

*T*aking care of yourself and developing a good self-care routine are imperative. Self-care means doing something therapeutic every day for yourself to improve your mental and physical health. You must make time for self-care every day, so it should be something you enjoy doing. This may sound hard at first because, well, it is a lot to commit to, but once you get into it, your self-care routine can quickly become your favorite part of the day.

The first step in developing a self-care routine is thinking about what you really enjoy doing. What brings you peace? What helps you feel centered and grounded? It doesn't have to be something big or time consuming; it just has to be something you really enjoy. Here are some examples:

- blasting your favorite song in the car on your way to work and singing along loudly
- taking a bubble bath at night
- practicing yoga
- taking a walk
- writing in a journal
- getting a massage
- going to the beach and watching the waves crash on the shore
- going for a hike
- painting your nails

Self-care should not be something you already do every day, such as checking Facebook for an hour. Nor does your self-care activity have to be consistent. Feel free to switch it up and do something different every day or every week, whatever feels right for you life. Activities that release energy are highly encouraged, like walking, riding a bike, practicing yoga, singing, dancing, and so on. But while physical activities are encouraged, they are certainly not required. Sometimes it's difficult for people with autoimmune diseases to be physically active due to pain and limitations in movement. If this is the case for you, your self-care routine might involve painting your nails, writing in a journal, or taking hot bubble baths (granted your joints are working well enough that you are able to get in and out of the tub). Make a list below of some ideas you have for your own self-care activities.

Self-Care Ideas

1. _____

2. _____

3. _____

4. _____

5. _____

6. _____

7. _____

8. _____

9. _____

10. _____

Now for the hard part—implementation of those ideas. Blocking out a set time every day doesn't work for everyone. If you are someone who has a job with consistent hours and a set schedule, working in a self-care routine may be a little easier. However, that is not the case for a lot of people, so on the following page is a self-care schedule you can use to take it day by day. It is meant to make your life easier, so if you struggle with the schedule provided, feel free to come up with your own ideas or your own way of using it.

Here is a suggestion for those interested. Next to the week heading, write the date range so you can keep track. For example, if you are starting your self-care routine on Monday, June 16, you would write *6/16–6/22* next to "week 1" so you know the dates that correspond with the weeks. In the blank boxes, write the time block you are setting aside for self-care on that day. For example, if you're on week one, in the box under Monday, you can write *5:00 p.m.–6:00 p.m.* so you know that this is the one hour you have identified on that day during which you have free time to dedicate to your self-care routine. It's good to plan ahead one or two weeks at a time so you can go through the week without having to think too much about fitting in self-care. I suggest spending an hour per day on yourself, but anything, even five minutes, is better than nothing.

If you can afford them, extra health care activities are beneficial. This can include getting a massage, receiving acupuncture or acupressure treatments—anything you can do once a month to rejuvenate your body. If this is something that is not really feasible given the mountain of medical bills you probably already have, see if you can recruit a friend, significant other, family member, or anyone else to give you a little back rub every once in a while. Some health insurance plans do cover massage therapy for people with chronic illnesses, so it's worth looking into. And never underestimate the power of a good, tight, long hug. Touch is a basic human need.

Below, you will find your self-care calendar.

Self-Care Routine Calendar

Month:	Monday	Tuesday	Wednesday	Thursday	Friday	Saturday	Sunday
Week 1							
Week 2							
Week 3							
Week 4							
Month:	Monday	Tuesday	Wednesday	Thursday	Friday	Saturday	Sunday
Week 1							
Week 2							
Week 3							
Week 4							
Month:	Monday	Tuesday	Wednesday	Thursday	Friday	Saturday	Sunday
Week 1							
Week 2							
Week 3							
Week 4							

Now you are ready to begin your self-care routine! Best of luck. Be well.

Conclusion

*M*azel tov—you've done it! You have worked your way through the steps, so sit back and take a nice deep breath. You should now have a clear picture in your mind of where you would like to see things with your health go, how to talk to professionals about getting there, and what you can do to take care of yourself in the meantime. These are all such important steps to taking control of your life and creating space for peace. It is my sincere hope that with time and your peer support network, you will find peace, comfort, hope, and stability. Take time to enjoy little things, and always tell the people you love that you love them. We are not always granted long lives, but that certainly doesn't mean we cannot live just as fully as anyone else. Know that you are not alone in this, and find comfort in those around you. Reach for help if you need it, and know that asking for help when you need it is one of the strongest things you can do.

With so much uncertainty caused by the complexity of autoimmune diseases, it helps to find stability in your life; it helps to feel centered and grounded. As much as you can, try to live a normal life. Travel when you're feeling well, set big goals for yourself, and make a dream board, or a poster that contains pictures of the things you want to accomplish in life, to hang in your room so every day when you wake up, you are inspired by the things you want to do most. Don't be afraid to ask for help opening bottles, tying shoes, buttoning shirts, or lifting a cup of coffee. People like feeling important and needed, so asking your coworkers to open a bottle of water for you every day most likely will make them feel good, too. Shalom.

About the Author

Cobi Silver, MSW, is a clinical crisis intervention social worker at three local hospitals in Washington. In addition, she has an autoimmune disease with co-occurring anxiety. The author has engaged in extensive research and review of scholarly articles related to autoimmune diseases, depression, and anxiety. She has also held focus groups about it and interviewed key informants. Her book draws from this research, as well as her own experience in the health care system. Silver received a bachelor of social work degree from Arizona State University and a master of social work degree from the University of Washington, Tacoma.

Cobi extends a special thank you to Katie Huckins who illustrated the cover of this book.

Bibliography

Aburizik, A., Dindo, L., Kaboli, P., Charlton, M., Dawn, K., & Turvey, C. (2013). A pilot randomized controlled trial of a depression and disease management program delivered by phone. *Journal of Affective Disorders, 151*(2), 769-774. doi:10.1016/j.jad.2013.06.028

Carr, F. N., Nicassio, P. M., Ishimori, M. L., Moldovan, I., Katsaros, E., Torralba, K., … Weisman, M. H. (2011). Depression predicts self-reported disease activity in systemic lupus erythematosus. *Lupus, 20*(1), 80-84. doi:10.1177/0961203310378672

Dantzer, R., O'Connor, J. C., Freund, G. G., Johnson, R. W., & Kelley, K. W. (2008). From inflammation to sickness and depression: When the immune system subjugates the brain. *Nature Reviews Neuroscience, 9*(1), 46-56. doi:10.1038/nrn2297

DeLuca, J., & Nocentini, U. (2011). Neuropsychological, medical and rehabilitative management of persons with multiple sclerosis. *Neurorehabilitation, 29*(3), 197-219. Retrieved from http://search.ebscohost.com/login.aspx?direct=true&db=a9h&AN=67655705&site=ehost-live

Gao, H., Sanders, E., Tieng, A. T., & Putterman, C. (2010). Sex and autoantibody titers determine the development of neuropsychiatric manifestations in lupus-prone mice. *Journal of Neuroimmunology, 229*(1), 112-122. doi:10.1016/j.jneuroim.2010.07.020

Isik, A., Koca, S., Ozturk, A., & Mermi, O. (2007). Anxiety and depression in patients with rheumatoid arthritis. *Clinical Rheumatology, 26*(6), 872-878. doi:10.1007/s10067-006-0407-y

Miwa, Y., Hosaka, M., Wakabayashi, K., Odai, T., Isozaki, T., Matsunawa, M., … Adachi, M. (2008). Rheumatoid arthritis patients with Sjögren's syndrome are more prone to depression than patients with rheumatoid arthritis or Sjögren's syndrome alone. *Current Rheumatology Reviews, 4*(1), 46-49. doi:10.2174/157339708783497973

Monaghan, S. M., Sharpe, L., Denton, F., Levy, J., Schrieber, L., & Sensky, T. (2007). Relationship between appearance and psychological distress in rheumatic diseases. *Arthritis & Rheumatism, 57*(2), 303-309. doi:10.1002/art.22553

Palagini, L., Mosca, M., Tani, C., Gemignani, A., Mauri, M., & Bombardieri, S. (2013). Depression and systemic lupus erythematosus: A systematic review. *Lupus, 22*(5), 409-416. doi:10.1177/0961203313477227

Rook, G. A. W., Raison, C. L., & Lowry, C. A. (2012). Can we vaccinate against depression? *Drug Discovery Today, 17*(9), 451-458. doi:10.1016/j.drudis.2012.03.018

Stoffel, M., Reis, D., Schwarz, D., & Schröder, A. (2013). Dimensions of coping in chronic pain patients: Factor analysis and cross-validation of the German version of the coping strategies questionnaire (CSQ-D). *Rehabilitation Psychology,* doi:10.1037/a0034358

Tjensvoll, A. B., Harboe, E., Gøransson, L. G., Beyer, M. K., Greve, O. J., Kvaløy, J. T., & Omdal, R. (2013). Headache in primary Sjögren's syndrome: A population-based retrospective cohort study. *European Journal of Neurology, 20*(3), 558-563. doi:10.1111/ene.12033

Zakeri, Z., Shakiba, M., Narouie, B., Mladkova, N., Ghasemi-Rad, M., & Khosravi, A. (2012). Prevalence of depression and depressive symptoms in patients with systemic lupus erythematosus: Iranian experience. *Rheumatology International, 32*(5), 1179-1187. doi:10.1007/s00296-010-1791-9

Zautra, A., Parrish, B., Puymbroeck, C., Tennen, H., Davis, M., Reich, J., & Irwin, M. (2007). Depression history, stress, and pain in rheumatoid arthritis patients. *Journal of Behavioral Medicine, 30*(3), 187-197. doi:10.1007/s10865-007-9097-4